THE COMPLETE HIGH BLOOD PRESSURE COOKBOOK FOR BEGINNERS

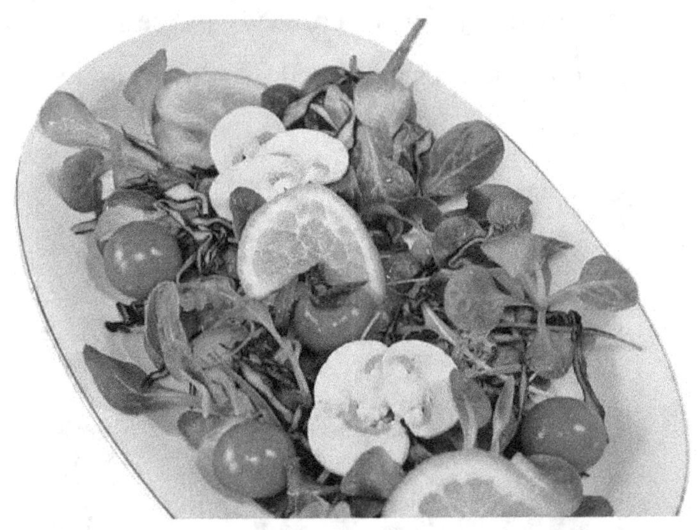

DR. VICKIE STOCK

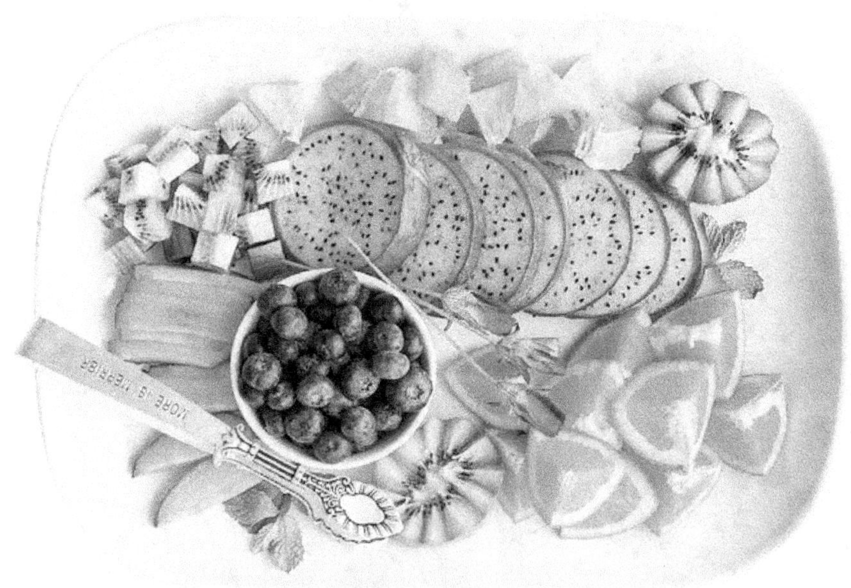

TABLE OF CONTENT

CHAPTER ONE: Understanding High Blood Pressure

Introduction to Blood Pressure

Blood pressure is a fundamental aspect of cardiovascular health, playing a crucial role in maintaining the body's equilibrium. It is a dynamic force exerted by the circulating blood against the walls of arteries as the heart pumps. Understanding blood pressure is essential, as it serves as a key indicator of cardiovascular well-being and can be a harbinger of potential health issues.

At its core, blood pressure is measured in millimeters of mercury (mmHg) and is expressed as two values: systolic and diastolic. The systolic pressure, the higher of the two values, represents the force exerted on arterial walls during the heart's contraction or pumping phase.

On the other hand, diastolic pressure, the lower value, signifies the force when the heart is in a relaxed or resting state between beats. The combination of these two measurements provides a comprehensive picture of the cardiovascular system's efficiency and resilience.

Blood pressure is dynamic, fluctuating throughout the day in response to various factors such as physical activity, stress, and even the time of day. Normal blood pressure typically falls within the range of 90/60 mmHg to 120/80 mmHg.

Deviations from this range, especially consistently elevated readings, may indicate hypertension or high blood pressure, a condition that demands attention and management.

The intricate mechanics of blood pressure involve the heart, blood vessels, and the blood itself. The heart, acting as a powerful muscular pump, propels oxygenated blood into the arteries, initiating a cascade of pressure changes.

Arteries, the vessels carrying blood away from the heart, respond to this force by expanding and contracting to accommodate the rhythmic flow. The delicate balance between these forces is essential for the proper circulation of blood to vital organs and tissues throughout the body.

Understanding blood pressure is not just about numbers on a monitor; it is about comprehending the delicate dance within the cardiovascular system that keeps our bodies nourished and functioning optimally.

As we delve deeper into this vital aspect of health, we will explore the significance of maintaining normal blood pressure, the factors influencing its fluctuations, and the potential consequences of disregarding its impact on overall well-being.

This journey into the intricacies of blood pressure will empower individuals, particularly beginners, to make informed choices for a heart-healthy life.

The Mechanics of Blood Pressure

The human circulatory system operates as a finely tuned network, with blood pressure serving as a vital indicator of its efficiency. To grasp the mechanics of blood pressure, one must delve into the intricate interplay between the heart, blood vessels, and the very substance that courses through our veins.

At the heart of this dynamic process is the muscular organ that acts as the body's primary pump—the heart. With each contraction, known as systole, the heart propels blood into the arteries, initiating a surge of pressure against their walls.

This force is measured as the systolic blood pressure, the higher value in the blood pressure reading. It represents the peak force exerted during the heart's contraction, signifying the moment when blood is forcefully ejected into the circulatory system.

As the heart relaxes between beats, a phase known as diastole, the pressure within the arteries decreases. This is reflected in the lower value of the blood pressure reading, known as diastolic blood pressure. The diastolic pressure represents the residual force within the arteries when the heart is at rest, awaiting the next contraction.

The blood vessels, particularly arteries, play a pivotal role in the mechanics of blood pressure. Arteries are not passive conduits; they exhibit elasticity and responsiveness to the pulsatile flow of blood.

During systole, arteries expand to accommodate the surge of blood, and during diastole, they contract to maintain a consistent pressure. This elasticity ensures a continuous and smooth flow of blood to various tissues and organs.

The composition of blood itself contributes to blood pressure dynamics. The blood volume, viscosity, and the concentration of red blood cells all influence the resistance encountered by blood as it travels through the vessels. The collective impact of these factors determines the overall resistance against which the heart must pump, affecting blood pressure levels.

Understanding the mechanics of blood pressure is essential for comprehending the body's cardiovascular health. Imbalances in this intricate system, such as persistent high blood pressure, can strain the heart and damage blood vessels over time, leading to serious health consequences.

By unraveling the mechanics of blood pressure, individuals gain insight into the inner workings of their circulatory system, empowering them to make informed lifestyle choices that promote heart health and overall well-being.

Normal vs. High Blood Pressure

Blood pressure, measured in millimeters of mercury (mmHg), is a crucial health parameter that serves as a barometer for cardiovascular well-being. Understanding the distinction between normal and high blood pressure is pivotal in recognizing potential health risks and adopting preventive measures.

Normal blood pressure falls within a specific range, typically around 90/60 mmHg to 120/80 mmHg. The first value, systolic pressure, reflects the force exerted on arterial walls during the heart's contraction, while the second value, diastolic pressure, signifies the force when the heart is at rest between beats.

These measurements indicate the optimal functioning of the circulatory system, ensuring that blood flows efficiently, supplying oxygen and nutrients to the body's organs and tissues.

In contrast, high blood pressure, also known as hypertension, occurs when the force of blood against the artery walls consistently exceeds the normal range.

Hypertension is often described in stages, ranging from Stage 1 (mild) to Stage 2 (moderate), and can pose significant health risks if left unmanaged. Persistent high blood pressure strains the heart, damages blood vessels, and increases the likelihood of developing serious conditions such as heart disease, stroke, and kidney problems.

Recognizing the difference between normal and high blood pressure involves paying attention to the numerical values and understanding the potential consequences of elevated readings.

While occasional fluctuations in blood pressure are normal in response to various factors like stress or physical activity, consistently high readings warrant attention and intervention.

The impact of high blood pressure extends beyond the cardiovascular system, affecting the kidneys, eyes, and other organs. Hypertension is often referred to as the "silent killer" because it may not present noticeable symptoms until significant damage has occurred. Regular monitoring of blood pressure, either at home or through healthcare providers, is essential for early detection and timely management.

Maintaining a healthy lifestyle is key to preventing high blood pressure. This includes a balanced diet low in sodium, regular physical activity, stress management, and avoiding tobacco and excessive alcohol consumption.

Understanding the distinction between normal and high blood pressure empowers individuals to take proactive steps in managing their cardiovascular health, reducing the risk of complications, and promoting a long and heart-healthy life.

Causes and Risk Factors

High blood pressure, or hypertension, is a multifaceted health condition influenced by a combination of genetic, lifestyle, and environmental factors.

Understanding the causes and risk factors is crucial for both preventing and managing this common yet potentially serious condition.

1. Genetics and Family History:

There is a genetic component to hypertension, meaning individuals with a family history of high blood pressure may have a higher predisposition. Specific genes that influence blood pressure regulation can be inherited, contributing to an increased risk of hypertension.

2. Age:

As individuals age, the risk of developing high blood pressure tends to increase. Arteries naturally lose some elasticity over time, and lifestyle factors accumulated throughout life may contribute to elevated blood pressure in older adults.

3. Lifestyle Choices:

Unhealthy lifestyle habits significantly contribute to high blood pressure.

Diets high in sodium, low in potassium, and lacking in fruits and vegetables can raise blood pressure. Sedentary lifestyles, lack of regular exercise, and excessive alcohol consumption are also modifiable risk factors.

4. Obesity: Being overweight or obese is a major risk factor for hypertension.

Excess body weight increases the workload on the heart, leading to higher blood pressure. Additionally, adipose tissue can produce substances that negatively impact blood vessel function and blood pressure regulation.

5. Tobacco Use:

Smoking and tobacco use have a direct and immediate effect on blood pressure. The chemicals in tobacco can damage blood vessels and accelerate the hardening of arteries, contributing to elevated blood pressure levels.

6. Chronic Stress:

Prolonged exposure to stress can contribute to high blood pressure. The body's response to stress involves the release of hormones that can temporarily raise blood pressure. Over time, chronic stress may lead to persistent hypertension.

7. Chronic Kidney Disease:

The kidneys play a crucial role in regulating blood pressure by managing fluid balance and filtering waste from the blood. Chronic kidney disease can disrupt these functions, leading to an increase in blood pressure.

8. Sleep Apnea: Sleep disorders, particularly obstructive sleep apnea, have been linked to hypertension.

Disrupted sleep patterns and inadequate oxygen intake during sleep can contribute to elevated blood pressure levels.

Recognizing these causes and risk factors allows individuals to make informed choices to mitigate their risk of developing high blood pressure.

Lifestyle modifications, regular health check-ups, and proactive management of contributing factors are essential steps in maintaining optimal cardiovascular health and preventing the complications associated with hypertension.

Why High Blood Pressure Matters

High blood pressure, or hypertension, is often referred to as the "silent killer" because it typically presents with no overt symptoms, yet its impact on overall health can be profound.

Understanding why high blood pressure matters is crucial for individuals to appreciate the significance of managing this condition and mitigating its potential consequences.

1. Increased Risk of Cardiovascular Diseases:

Persistent high blood pressure places immense strain on the heart and blood vessels, increasing the risk of serious cardiovascular diseases.

Hypertension is a major contributor to conditions such as coronary artery disease, heart failure, and stroke.

The elevated force of blood against arterial walls can lead to the gradual accumulation of damage, ultimately compromising the cardiovascular system's functionality.

2. Damage to Blood Vessels:

The continuous pressure exerted by high blood pressure can damage the delicate inner lining of blood vessels. This damage, often referred to as endothelial dysfunction, can result in the formation of plaques, narrowing the arteries and impeding blood flow. Over time, this can lead to atherosclerosis, a condition associated with an increased risk of heart attacks and strokes.

3. Strain on the Heart:

The heart works harder to pump blood against elevated resistance in hypertensive individuals. This increased workload can lead to the thickening of the heart muscle, a condition known as left ventricular hypertrophy. Left untreated, this can impair the heart's ability to pump efficiently, leading to heart failure.

4. Kidney Damage:

The kidneys play a crucial role in regulating blood pressure. Chronic hypertension can damage the kidneys' blood vessels and compromise their ability to filter waste from the blood. This, in turn, can contribute to kidney disease or failure.

5. Vision Impairment:

Hypertension can adversely affect the blood vessels in the eyes, potentially leading to vision problems or even blindness. Conditions such as hypertensive retinopathy can result from the damage inflicted on the small blood vessels in the retina.

6. Cognitive Decline and Dementia:

Research suggests a link between high blood pressure and an increased risk of cognitive decline and dementia, including Alzheimer's disease. The compromised blood flow to the brain associated with hypertension may contribute to these cognitive impairments.

7. Increased Risk During Pregnancy:

High blood pressure during pregnancy, known as gestational hypertension or preeclampsia, can pose risks to both the mother and the developing fetus. Complications may include premature birth, low birth weight, and long-term health issues for the baby.

Understanding why high blood pressure matters underscores the importance of regular monitoring, lifestyle modifications, and, if necessary, medical interventions.

By actively managing blood pressure, individuals can significantly reduce their risk of developing severe health complications and enhance their overall well-being. Prioritizing heart health is a proactive step towards a longer, healthier life.

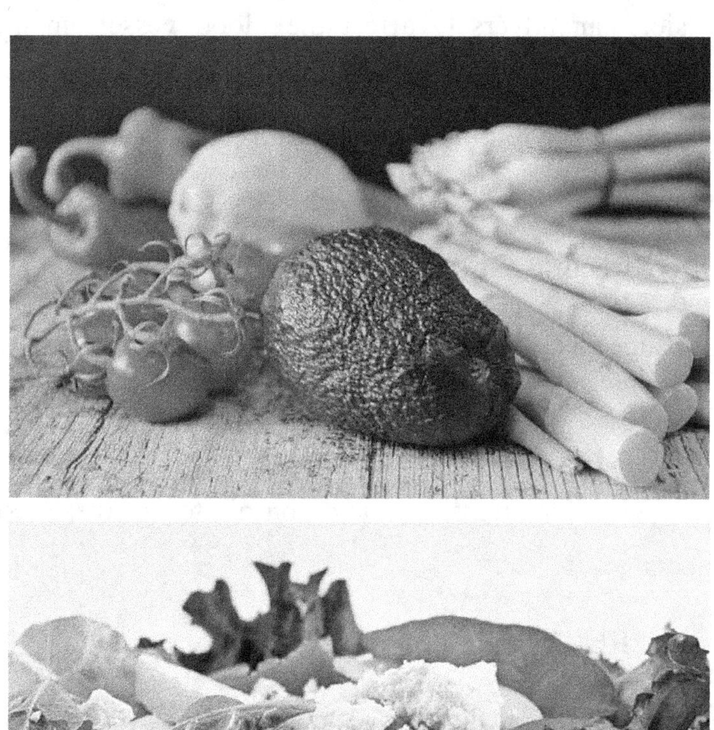

CHAPTER TWO: Diagnosing and monitoring High blood Pressure

The Importance of Regular Blood Pressure Checks

Regular blood pressure checks play a pivotal role in maintaining overall health and preventing the silent threat of hypertension. Blood pressure, the force of blood against the walls of arteries, is a critical indicator of cardiovascular well-being.

Understanding the importance of monitoring blood pressure regularly is essential for early detection, prevention, and effective management of high blood pressure.

First and foremost, regular blood pressure checks serve as a proactive measure in identifying potential health risks. Hypertension, often referred to as the "silent killer," may not present obvious symptoms in its early stages.

Routine monitoring allows individuals and healthcare professionals to catch elevated blood pressure levels before they escalate into more severe health issues. Early detection facilitates timely interventions, minimizing the risk of complications such as heart disease, stroke, and kidney problems.

Additionally, blood pressure fluctuations can occur due to various factors, including stress, diet, and physical activity. Regular monitoring provides valuable insights into these patterns, enabling individuals to make informed lifestyle choices. By identifying triggers or contributors to high blood pressure, individuals can adopt healthier habits, such as incorporating exercise, reducing salt intake, and managing stress, to maintain optimal blood pressure levels.

Regular blood pressure checks are particularly crucial for individuals with known risk factors for hypertension, such as age, family history, or certain medical conditions. Consistent monitoring empowers both individuals and healthcare professionals to tailor treatment plans based on real-time data, ensuring personalized and effective management strategies.

Moreover, routine blood pressure checks contribute to a culture of preventive healthcare. Waiting for symptoms to manifest before seeking medical attention can lead to delayed diagnosis and treatment. Regular monitoring encourages a proactive mindset, promoting wellness and preventing the progression of potential health issues.

Technology advancements have made blood pressure monitoring more accessible than ever. Home blood pressure monitors allow individuals to track their readings conveniently, promoting a more active role in their healthcare.

However, it's essential to complement self-monitoring with periodic professional check-ups to ensure accuracy and receive expert guidance on managing blood pressure effectively.

How Blood Pressure is Measured

Measuring blood pressure is a fundamental aspect of cardiovascular health assessment, providing crucial insights into the force exerted by blood on the walls of arteries.

Understanding the process of blood pressure measurement involves familiarity with the tools used, the significance of blood pressure readings, and the factors influencing accurate assessment.

Blood pressure is typically measured using a sphygmomanometer, an inflatable cuff, and a stethoscope. The process involves wrapping the cuff around the upper arm, positioning it over the brachial artery.

The cuff is then inflated to temporarily cut off blood flow. As the cuff gradually deflates, a healthcare professional or an automated device listens for the characteristic sounds of blood flow using the stethoscope or digital sensors.

Blood pressure readings are expressed as two values: systolic pressure over diastolic pressure. The systolic pressure represents the force when the heart contracts, pushing blood into the arteries, while diastolic pressure indicates the force when the heart is at rest between beats.

The unit of measurement is millimeters of mercury (mmHg). For example, a blood pressure reading of 120/80 mmHg means a systolic pressure of 120 mmHg and a diastolic pressure of 80 mmHg.

Understanding these two values is essential as they convey distinct information about the cardiovascular system. Elevated systolic pressure may signify increased cardiac workload, while elevated diastolic pressure may indicate arterial stiffness. Both values together provide a comprehensive picture of overall blood pressure health.

Several factors can influence blood pressure measurements, including the individual's posture, activity level, and emotional state. To account for these variables, it is recommended to measure blood pressure in a relaxed, seated position after a few minutes of rest. Multiple readings over different sessions help establish a more accurate baseline and account for variations.

Advancements in technology have introduced automated blood pressure monitors for convenient self-monitoring at home. These devices use oscillometric methods to measure blood pressure, eliminating the need for a stethoscope.

While home monitoring is valuable for tracking trends, it's crucial to complement it with periodic professional measurements to ensure accuracy and address any concerns promptly.

Understanding how blood pressure is measured is essential for interpreting cardiovascular health. Regular and accurate measurements offer valuable information for assessing risk, guiding interventions, and promoting overall well-being.

Understanding Blood Pressure Readings

Interpreting blood pressure readings is key to assessing cardiovascular health and understanding potential risks. Blood pressure readings consist of two numbers, with each providing essential information about the heart's pumping action and the resistance of arteries. Grasping the significance of these readings empowers individuals to take an active role in their health and make informed decisions regarding lifestyle and medical interventions.

The first number in a blood pressure reading is the systolic pressure, representing the force of blood against arterial walls when the heart contracts during a heartbeat. It is the higher of the two numbers and reflects the maximum pressure in the arteries.

Systolic pressure is crucial for assessing the heart's ability to pump blood effectively throughout the body.

The second number is the diastolic pressure, representing the force of blood when the heart is at rest between beats. This number is the lower of the two and reflects the minimum pressure in the arteries. Diastolic pressure is vital for evaluating the overall resistance in the arteries, indicating how well blood vessels are relaxing and allowing blood to flow. Blood pressure readings are expressed in millimeters of mercury (mmHg), with normal readings falling around 120/80 mmHg. However, the American Heart Association classifies blood pressure ranges differently:

Normal: Systolic <120 mmHg and Diastolic <80 mmHg

Elevated: Systolic 120-129 mmHg and Diastolic <80 mmHg

Hypertension Stage 1: Systolic 130-139 mmHg or Diastolic 80-89 mmHg

Hypertension Stage 2: Systolic ≥140 mmHg or Diastolic ≥90 mmHg

Hypertensive Crisis: Systolic >180 mmHg and/or Diastolic >120 mmHg

Understanding these categories helps individuals and healthcare professionals identify potential risks and formulate appropriate interventions. Consistent monitoring is crucial, as variations in readings can occur due to factors such as stress, physical activity, or underlying health conditions.

It's important to note that a single high reading does not necessarily indicate hypertension. Trends over time and multiple readings provide a more accurate assessment. Lifestyle modifications, including a healthy diet, regular exercise, stress management, and medication when necessary, can effectively manage and lower blood pressure.

Monitoring Blood Pressure at Home

Home blood pressure monitoring has become an invaluable tool in managing cardiovascular health, offering individuals the convenience of regular assessments and contributing to proactive healthcare practices.

This approach empowers people to take an active role in monitoring their blood pressure, leading to early detection of abnormalities and enabling timely interventions.

Understanding the benefits and best practices of monitoring blood pressure at home is crucial for effective self-care.

One of the primary advantages of home blood pressure monitoring is the ability to measure blood pressure in a familiar and relaxed environment.

This contrasts with the potential stress or anxiety associated with clinical settings, often referred to as "white coat syndrome," which can lead to inaccurate readings. By taking measurements at home, individuals obtain a more accurate reflection of their day-to-day blood pressure levels.

Choosing an appropriate home blood pressure monitor is essential. Automatic digital monitors are popular for their ease of use and accuracy. These devices typically include an arm cuff that inflates automatically, providing digital readings displayed on a screen. Wrist monitors are also available but may be less accurate and sensitive to body position.

Consistency is key when monitoring blood pressure at home. It's recommended to measure blood pressure at the same time each day, usually in the morning and evening, and to follow a standardized procedure. This involves sitting quietly for a few minutes before the measurement, supporting the arm at heart level, and avoiding caffeine, exercise, or smoking in the 30 minutes preceding the reading.

Recording and tracking blood pressure readings over time is essential for identifying trends and sharing information with healthcare professionals. Many home monitors come equipped with memory features or can sync with smartphone apps, allowing for easy tracking and sharing of data during medical appointments.

While home monitoring provides valuable insights, it's crucial to complement it with periodic professional measurements. Healthcare professionals can verify the accuracy of home readings, offer guidance on interpretation, and adjust treatment plans accordingly.

Home blood pressure monitoring is particularly beneficial for individuals with hypertension, those on medication, or those at risk of developing high blood pressure. It promotes a sense of responsibility for one's health and facilitates early intervention, reducing the risk of complications associated with uncontrolled hypertension.

High blood pressure, or hypertension, is often dubbed the "silent killer" due to its asymptomatic nature in its early stages. However, as the condition progresses, certain signs may emerge, signaling the need for immediate attention and medical intervention.

Recognizing symptoms of high blood pressure is crucial for early detection, effective management, and the prevention of potential complications.

One of the most concerning aspects of hypertension is its subtlety, with many individuals unaware of their elevated blood pressure until complications arise. As blood pressure increases, some people may experience persistent headaches, particularly at the back of the head. This can be an indication of heightened pressure within the blood vessels of the brain.

Visual disturbances, such as blurred or double vision, may also manifest in individuals with uncontrolled high blood pressure.

This occurs due to the impact of increased pressure on the small blood vessels in the eyes, highlighting the intricate connection between hypertension and organ damage.

Fatigue and difficulty in concentrating are common symptoms associated with high blood pressure. Reduced blood flow to vital organs, including the brain, can lead to feelings of lethargy and diminished cognitive function. If these symptoms persist, they warrant thorough investigation to determine their underlying cause.

Shortness of breath and chest pain are alarming symptoms that should never be ignored. Uncontrolled high blood pressure can strain the heart, leading to the development of cardiovascular issues such as coronary artery disease or heart failure. Individuals experiencing chest pain or difficulty breathing should seek immediate medical attention, as these symptoms may indicate a potential cardiac event.

It's crucial to note that symptoms of high blood pressure can vary from person to person, and some individuals may not experience any noticeable signs. Regular blood pressure monitoring, especially for those with risk factors, is paramount for early detection and prevention.

Given the potential severity of hypertension, routine check-ups with healthcare professionals are vital. Blood pressure measurements during these visits help identify elevated readings and prompt further investigations. Lifestyle modifications, including dietary changes, regular exercise, stress management, and, if necessary, medication, can effectively manage high blood pressure and reduce the risk of complications.

CHAPTER THREE: Lifestyle Changes for Managing High blood Pressure

Dietary Approaches to Lowering Blood Pressure

Maintaining a healthy diet is a cornerstone of managing high blood pressure, providing individuals with a powerful and proactive means to take control of their cardiovascular health. The right dietary choices can play a pivotal role in reducing blood pressure and minimizing the risk of associated complications. Here are key dietary approaches that beginners can adopt to effectively lower blood pressure.

1. Embrace the DASH Diet:

The Dietary Approaches to Stop Hypertension (DASH) diet has garnered widespread recognition for its efficacy in reducing blood pressure. Emphasizing fruits, vegetables, lean proteins, and whole grains, the DASH diet promotes a well-balanced and nutrient-rich approach to eating.

By minimizing sodium intake and encouraging the consumption of potassium-rich foods, such as bananas, oranges, and leafy greens, individuals can help regulate blood pressure levels.

2. Reduce Sodium Intake:

Excessive sodium intake is a known contributor to elevated blood pressure.

Processed and packaged foods are often high in sodium, so opting for fresh, whole foods and cooking at home allows better control over salt content. Reading food labels diligently and choosing low-sodium alternatives can significantly impact overall sodium consumption.

3. Increase Potassium-Rich Foods:

Potassium acts as a counterbalance to sodium, helping to regulate fluid balance and relax blood vessel walls. Incorporating potassium-rich foods into the diet, such as sweet potatoes, spinach, and bananas, can enhance the body's ability to maintain a healthy blood pressure. However, it's essential to strike a balance, as excessive potassium intake can also have adverse effects, particularly for those with kidney-related issues.

4. Emphasize Magnesium and Calcium:

Magnesium and calcium are essential minerals that contribute to cardiovascular health. Foods like nuts, seeds, leafy greens, and dairy products are excellent sources of these minerals. Including a variety of these foods in the diet not only supports blood pressure regulation but also promotes overall heart health.

5. Adopt a Heart-Healthy Lifestyle:

Beyond specific dietary choices, adopting a heart-healthy lifestyle complements efforts to lower blood pressure. This includes maintaining a healthy weight, engaging in regular physical activity, moderating alcohol consumption, and avoiding tobacco. These lifestyle factors collectively contribute to overall cardiovascular well-being.

A well-rounded dietary approach involves not only reducing sodium but also embracing nutrient-dense foods that support heart health. By incorporating these dietary strategies into daily life, beginners can take meaningful steps towards managing and lowering their blood pressure effectively. Always consult with a healthcare professional for personalized advice tailored to individual health needs and conditions.

Importance of Regular Exercise for Managing Blood Pressure

Regular exercise is a cornerstone in the management of high blood pressure, offering a natural and effective means to promote cardiovascular health. Engaging in physical activity not only helps lower blood pressure but also contributes to overall well-being. Here's a closer look at the importance of regular exercise for individuals looking to manage their blood pressure levels.

1. Improved Cardiovascular Health:

Exercise is a powerful tool for strengthening the heart and improving overall cardiovascular health. As individuals engage in regular physical activity, the heart becomes more efficient at pumping blood, leading to a reduction in the force exerted on the arteries. This, in turn, can contribute to lower blood pressure levels.

2. Weight Management:

Maintaining a healthy weight is crucial for blood pressure regulation. Regular exercise helps individuals achieve and sustain a healthy body weight by burning calories and promoting fat loss. By reducing excess body weight, the workload on the heart is decreased, leading to improved blood pressure control.

3. Enhanced Blood Vessel Function:

Physical activity stimulates the production of nitric oxide, a compound that helps dilate blood vessels, promoting improved blood flow. This dilation of blood vessels reduces resistance, making it easier for blood to circulate throughout the body. The enhanced flexibility of blood vessels contributes to better blood pressure management.

4. Stress Reduction:

Chronic stress can contribute to elevated blood pressure. Exercise serves as a powerful stress-reliever, triggering the release of endorphins—feel-good hormones that act as natural mood elevators. Regular physical activity helps manage stress levels, creating a positive impact on both mental and cardiovascular health.

5. Consistent Blood Pressure Regulation:

Engaging in regular exercise establishes a consistent pattern of blood pressure regulation. While acute bouts of physical activity may lead to temporary increases in blood pressure, the long-term effects are overwhelmingly positive. Regular exercise conditions the cardiovascular system, leading to sustained improvements in blood pressure over time.

6. Type 2 Diabetes Prevention:

Individuals with diabetes are at an increased risk of developing high blood pressure. Regular exercise not only aids in blood pressure control but also plays a vital role in preventing and managing type 2 diabetes. By improving insulin sensitivity and glucose metabolism, exercise contributes to overall metabolic health.

The importance of regular exercise in managing blood pressure cannot be overstated. It offers a holistic approach to cardiovascular health, encompassing weight management, improved blood vessel function, stress reduction, and consistent blood pressure regulation.

Stress Management Techniques

Chronic stress has been identified as a significant contributor to high blood pressure, making stress management a crucial component of a comprehensive approach to cardiovascular health.

Implementing effective stress management techniques not only promotes mental well-being but also aids in maintaining optimal blood pressure levels. Here are key strategies for managing stress to support blood pressure control:

1. Mindfulness Meditation:

Mindfulness meditation involves focusing on the present moment without judgment. By practicing mindfulness, individuals can cultivate a sense of calm and reduce the impact of stress on both the mind and body. Studies have shown that regular mindfulness meditation can contribute to lower blood pressure levels over time.

2. Deep Breathing Exercises:

Deep breathing exercises, such as diaphragmatic breathing or paced respiration, activate the body's relaxation response. By slowing down the breathing rate and promoting deep inhalation and exhalation, these exercises help reduce stress hormones and lower blood pressure. Incorporating deep breathing into daily routines can provide immediate relief during stressful situations.

3. Regular Physical Activity:

Exercise not only benefits the cardiovascular system but also serves as a powerful stress-reduction tool. Physical activity stimulates the release of endorphins, the body's natural mood lifters, and helps dissipate accumulated tension.

Engaging in activities like walking, jogging, or yoga on a regular basis can contribute to long-term stress management.

4. Time Management and Prioritization:

Stress often arises from feeling overwhelmed by a multitude of tasks. Effective time management and prioritization can help individuals regain a sense of control.

Breaking tasks into smaller, more manageable steps, setting realistic goals, and learning to delegate when necessary can alleviate the pressures that contribute to stress.

5. Social Support and Connection:

Maintaining strong social connections is crucial for emotional well-being. Sharing concerns and seeking support from friends, family, or support groups can provide a valuable outlet for stress relief.

Positive social interactions trigger the release of oxytocin, a hormone that promotes feelings of bonding and reduces stress.

6. Adequate Sleep:

Quality sleep plays a vital role in stress management. Chronic sleep deprivation can elevate stress hormones and contribute to increased blood pressure. Establishing a regular sleep routine, creating a comfortable sleep environment, and practicing relaxation techniques before bedtime are essential for promoting restful sleep.

7. Relaxation Techniques:

Incorporating relaxation techniques, such as progressive muscle relaxation or guided imagery, can effectively reduce stress levels. These methods help relax tense muscles and redirect the mind's focus away from stressors, promoting a state of physical and mental calmness.

Quitting Smoking and Limiting Alcohol Intake

Making lifestyle changes by quitting smoking and moderating alcohol intake are paramount for individuals aiming to manage their blood pressure effectively.

Both smoking and excessive alcohol consumption have direct and adverse effects on cardiovascular health, contributing to elevated blood pressure and increasing the risk of related complications. Here's a closer look at the importance of quitting smoking and limiting alcohol intake for blood pressure control.

1. Smoking Cessation:

Quitting smoking is one of the most impactful steps individuals can take to improve their cardiovascular health. The harmful chemicals in tobacco smoke not only damage blood vessels but also elevate heart rate, leading to increased blood pressure.

Upon quitting, the body begins to repair itself, and blood pressure often starts to decline within weeks.

Successful smoking cessation not only benefits blood pressure control but also reduces the risk of heart disease and stroke.

2. Nicotine Replacement Therapy (NRT):

For those struggling to quit smoking, nicotine replacement therapy (NRT) can be a valuable aid. NRT products, such as patches, gum, or lozenges, provide controlled doses of nicotine without the harmful substances found in cigarettes. This can help manage withdrawal symptoms and increase the likelihood of successfully quitting.

3. Alcohol Moderation:

While moderate alcohol consumption may have some cardiovascular benefits, excessive drinking can lead to hypertension and other heart-related issues.

The American Heart Association defines moderate drinking as up to one drink per day for women and up to two drinks per day for men. Consuming alcohol within these limits may have protective effects on the heart, but exceeding them can contribute to elevated blood pressure.

4. Understanding Standard Drink Sizes:

To moderate alcohol intake effectively, it's essential to understand standard drink sizes. A standard drink is generally defined as 14 grams of pure alcohol, equivalent to about 5 ounces of wine, 12 ounces of beer, or 1.5 ounces of distilled spirits. Monitoring and limiting alcohol intake based on these measurements is key to maintaining a healthy balance.

5. Alcohol-Free Days:

Incorporating alcohol-free days into the week can help reset drinking patterns and promote overall health.

This practice allows the body time to recover and reduces the cumulative impact of alcohol on blood pressure. Choosing non-alcoholic alternatives during these periods supports the goal of moderation.

6. Seeking Professional Support:

For individuals struggling to quit smoking or moderate alcohol intake, seeking professional support is crucial. Healthcare providers can offer guidance, recommend cessation programs, and provide resources to address the physical and psychological aspects of addiction.

Developing Healthy Sleep Habits

Establishing and maintaining healthy sleep habits is a crucial aspect of overall well-being, particularly for individuals managing high blood pressure.

Quality sleep plays a pivotal role in regulating various physiological functions, including blood pressure.

Here's an exploration of the importance of developing healthy sleep habits and their impact on blood pressure.

1. Prioritize Consistent Sleep Schedule:

Maintaining a consistent sleep schedule is essential for regulating the body's internal clock. Going to bed and waking up at the same time each day helps synchronize circadian rhythms, promoting more restorative sleep. Erratic sleep patterns can disrupt these rhythms, potentially contributing to elevated blood pressure.

2. Create a Relaxing Bedtime Routine:

Establishing a calming bedtime routine signals to the body that it's time to wind down. Activities such as reading a book, taking a warm bath, or practicing relaxation exercises can help relax the mind and body, facilitating a smoother transition into sleep. Avoiding stimulating activities, like screen time, close to bedtime is also beneficial.

3. Ensure a Comfortable Sleep Environment:

Optimal sleep requires a comfortable and conducive sleep environment. This includes a supportive mattress and pillows, as well as a cool, dark, and quiet room.

Creating a sleep-conducive atmosphere enhances the likelihood of restful and uninterrupted sleep, positively impacting blood pressure regulation.

4. Limit Stimulants and Heavy Meals Before Bed:

Caffeine and nicotine are stimulants that can interfere with the ability to fall asleep. It's advisable to avoid consuming these substances close to bedtime. '

Additionally, heavy meals before bed can cause discomfort and indigestion, potentially disrupting sleep. Opting for lighter evening meals can contribute to a more restful night.

5. Regular Physical Activity:

Regular physical activity not only benefits cardiovascular health but also promotes better sleep. Engaging in moderate-intensity exercise, such as walking or jogging, can contribute to improved sleep quality. However, it's important to complete exercise sessions at least a few hours before bedtime to avoid potential sleep disruption.

6. Limit Naps and Manage Stress:

While short naps can be refreshing, extended or irregular napping during the day can interfere with nighttime sleep. If needed, limit naps to 20-30 minutes. Additionally, managing stress through techniques such as meditation, deep breathing, or yoga can enhance the ability to cope with daily challenges, promoting a more relaxed state conducive to quality sleep.

7. Seek Professional Guidance for Persistent Sleep Issues:

If sleep problems persist, seeking guidance from healthcare professionals is crucial. Conditions such as sleep apnea, insomnia, or restless leg syndrome can impact sleep quality and, in turn, influence blood pressure. Addressing underlying sleep disorders can lead to more effective blood pressure management.

High Blood Pressure Foods to eat and Foods to Avoid

Maintaining a heart-healthy diet is essential for managing high blood pressure. Choosing nutrient-rich foods can contribute to better blood pressure control and overall cardiovascular health. Here are some foods to include in a high blood pressure-friendly diet:

- Leafy Greens: Leafy greens such as spinach, kale, and Swiss chard are rich in potassium, a mineral that helps balance sodium levels and promote blood vessel health.
- Berries: Berries like blueberries, strawberries, and raspberries contain antioxidants known as flavonoids, which have been linked to lower blood pressure levels.
- Oats: Oats are a good source of beta-glucans, a type of soluble fiber that can help reduce cholesterol levels and support heart health.

- ➤ Bananas: Bananas are high in potassium, a mineral that helps regulate blood pressure by balancing the effects of sodium.

- ➤ Fatty Fish: Fatty fish such as salmon, mackerel, and trout are rich in omega-3 fatty acids, which have been associated with lower blood pressure and improved heart health.

- ➤ Beets: Beets contain nitrates, which can help dilate blood vessels and improve blood flow, potentially leading to lower blood pressure.

- ➤ Garlic: Garlic has been linked to potential blood pressure-lowering effects, and incorporating it into meals can add flavor and potential health benefits.

- ➤ Nuts and Seeds: Almonds, walnuts, chia seeds, and flaxseeds are good sources of potassium, magnesium, and fiber, all of which contribute to heart health.

- ➤ Low-Fat Dairy: Low-fat or fat-free dairy products, such as yogurt and milk, provide calcium and protein without the saturated fats found in full-fat options.

- ➤ Olive Oil: Olive oil is a heart-healthy monounsaturated fat that can be used as a substitute for less healthy cooking oils.

Including a variety of these foods in a well-balanced diet can contribute to a heart-healthy lifestyle and support efforts to manage high blood pressure.

High Blood Pressure: Foods to Avoid

When managing high blood pressure, it's crucial to be mindful of certain foods that can contribute to elevated blood pressure and overall cardiovascular risk. Here are foods to limit or avoid in a high blood pressure diet:

- ➤ Processed and Canned Foods: These often contain high levels of sodium, contributing to water retention and increased blood pressure. Opt for fresh or minimally processed alternatives.
- ➤ Salted Snacks: Chips, pretzels, and other salted snacks can be major sources of sodium, negatively impacting blood pressure levels.
- ➤ Canned Soups and Broths: These commonly have high sodium content. Choosing low-sodium or making homemade versions allows for better control of salt intake.
- ➤ Processed Meats: Cold cuts, bacon, sausage, and other processed meats are high in sodium and may contain unhealthy saturated fats.
- ➤ Frozen Dinners: Convenience meals often contain excessive salt. Preparing fresh meals at home with herbs and spices for flavoring is a healthier option.
- ➤ Canned Vegetables with Added Salt: Opt for fresh or frozen vegetables without added salt to control sodium intake.

➢ Sugary Drinks: High sugar intake may contribute to weight gain and increased blood pressure. Choose water, herbal tea, or other low-calorie beverages.

➢ Excessive Caffeine: While moderate caffeine intake is generally acceptable, excessive amounts can lead to a temporary spike in blood pressure. Monitor coffee and energy drink consumption.

➢ High-Fat Dairy: Full-fat dairy products can contribute to unhealthy cholesterol levels. Choose low-fat or fat-free options for a heart-healthy alternative.

➢ Highly Processed and Fried Foods: These often contain unhealthy fats and may contribute to weight gain and cardiovascular issues.

Being mindful of these foods and making informed choices can significantly contribute to blood pressure management and overall heart health.

Always consult with healthcare professionals for personalized dietary recommendations based on individual health conditions.

CHAPTER FOUR: High Blood Pressure Recipes

Breakfast Recipes:

1. Oatmeal with Berries and Nuts

Ingredients:

- 1/2 cup rolled oats
- 1 cup mixed berries (strawberries, blueberries, raspberries)
- 2 tablespoons chopped nuts (walnuts or almonds)
- 1 teaspoon honey
- 1 cup low-fat milk

Instructions:

- Cook oats according to package instructions.
- Top with mixed berries, chopped nuts, and a drizzle of honey.
- Serve with a cup of low-fat milk.

Health Benefits:

- Oats contain beta-glucans, which may help lower cholesterol.

Preparation Time: 10 minutes

2. Avocado Toast with Tomato and Spinach

Ingredients:

- 1 slice whole-grain bread

- ➢ 1/2 ripe avocado
- ➢ 1 small tomato, sliced
- ➢ Handful of fresh spinach
- ➢ Salt and pepper to taste

Instructions:

- ➢ Toast the bread slice.
- ➢ Mash the avocado and spread it over the toast.
- ➢ Top with sliced tomato and fresh spinach.
- ➢ Season with salt and pepper.

Health Benefits:

- ➢ Avocado provides heart-healthy monounsaturated fats.

Preparation Time: 5 minutes

3. Greek Yogurt Parfait

Ingredients:

- ➢ 1 cup low-fat Greek yogurt
- ➢ 1/2 cup mixed berries
- ➢ 2 tablespoons granola
- ➢ 1 tablespoon honey

Instructions:

- ➢ In a glass, layer Greek yogurt, mixed berries, and granola.
- ➢ Repeat the layers.

➢ Drizzle honey on top.

Health Benefits:

➢ Greek yogurt is rich in potassium, which can help balance sodium levels.

Preparation Time: 5 minutes

4. Spinach and Feta Omelette

Ingredients:

➢ 2 large eggs
➢ Handful of fresh spinach, chopped
➢ 2 tablespoons feta cheese, crumbled
➢ 1/4 cup cherry tomatoes, halved
➢ Salt and pepper to taste

Instructions:

➢ Whisk eggs in a bowl and season with salt and pepper.
➢ In a non-stick pan, sauté spinach until wilted.
➢ Pour whisked eggs over spinach, add feta and cherry tomatoes.
➢ Cook until eggs are set, then fold in half.

Health Benefits:

➢ Spinach is rich in potassium and feta provides calcium.

Preparation Time: 10 minutes

5. Quinoa Breakfast Bowl

Ingredients:

- 1/2 cup cooked quinoa
- 1/4 cup sliced almonds
- 1/2 banana, sliced
- 1 tablespoon chia seeds
- 1/4 cup unsweetened almond milk

Instructions:

- In a bowl, combine quinoa, sliced almonds, banana, and chia seeds.
- Pour almond milk over the mixture.
- Stir well before serving.

Health Benefits:

- Quinoa contains protein and essential amino acids.

Preparation Time: 15 minutes (including quinoa preparation)

6. Chia Seed Pudding with Mango

Ingredients:

- 2 tablespoons chia seeds
- 1/2 cup unsweetened almond milk
- 1/2 teaspoon vanilla extract
- 1/2 mango, diced

Instructions:

> - Mix chia seeds, almond milk, and vanilla extract in a bowl.
> - Refrigerate overnight or for at least 3 hours.
> - Top with diced mango before serving.

Health Benefits:

> - Chia seeds are rich in omega-3 fatty acids and fiber.

Preparation Time: 5 minutes (plus chilling time)

7. Whole Wheat Pancakes with Blueberry Compote

Ingredients:

> - 1 cup whole wheat flour
> - 1 tablespoon baking powder
> - 1 tablespoon honey
> - 1 cup almond milk
> - 1 cup blueberries (fresh or frozen)

Instructions:

> - In a bowl, whisk together flour, baking powder, honey, and almond milk.
> - Heat a griddle or non-stick pan and pour 1/4 cup of batter for each pancake.
> - Cook until bubbles form, flip, and cook until golden.

> In a saucepan, simmer blueberries until they break down to make a compote.

Health Benefits:

> Whole wheat provides more fiber, and blueberries are rich in antioxidants.

Preparation Time: 15 minutes

8. Salmon and Avocado Bagel

Ingredients:

> 1 whole-grain bagel, toasted
> 2 ounces smoked salmon
> 1/2 avocado, sliced
> 1 tablespoon cream cheese
> Capers and fresh dill for garnish

Instructions:

> Spread cream cheese on the toasted bagel halves.
> Top with smoked salmon, avocado slices, capers, and fresh dill.

Health Benefits:

> Salmon provides omega-3 fatty acids, beneficial for heart health.

Preparation Time: 10 minutes

9. Sweet Potato Hash with Poached Eggs

Ingredients:

- ➢ 1 sweet potato, grated
- ➢ 1 tablespoon olive oil
- ➢ 2 eggs, poached
- ➢ Salt and pepper to taste
- ➢ Fresh parsley for garnish

Instructions:

- ➢ Sauté grated sweet potato in olive oil until cooked and slightly crispy.
- ➢ Poach eggs and place them on top of the sweet potato hash.
- ➢ Season with salt, pepper, and garnish with fresh parsley.

Health Benefits:

- ➢ Sweet potatoes are rich in potassium and fiber.

Preparation Time: 15 minutes

10. Berry and Spinach Smoothie Bowl

Ingredients:

- ➢ 1 cup spinach leaves
- ➢ 1/2 cup mixed berries (strawberries, blueberries, raspberries)

- ➤ 1/2 banana
- ➤ 1/2 cup low-fat Greek yogurt
- ➤ 1 tablespoon chia seeds

Instructions:

- ➤ Blend spinach, berries, banana, and Greek yogurt until smooth.
- ➤ Pour into a bowl and top with chia seeds.

Health Benefits:

- ➤ Spinach contributes to overall heart health, and berries offer antioxidants.

Preparation Time: 5 minutes

11. Brown Rice Breakfast Bowl

Ingredients:

- ➤ 1/2 cup cooked brown rice
- ➤ 1/4 cup sliced almonds
- ➤ 1/2 apple, diced
- ➤ 1 tablespoon honey
- ➤ 1/2 cup skim milk

Instructions:

- ➤ Combine brown rice, sliced almonds, diced apple, and honey in a bowl.

➤ Pour skim milk over the mixture.

Health Benefits:

➤ Brown rice is a whole grain rich in fiber, and almonds provide healthy fats.

Preparation Time: 10 minutes (including rice preparation)

12. Green Tea Smoothie

Ingredients:

➤ 1 cup brewed green tea, cooled
➤ 1/2 cup pineapple chunks
➤ 1/2 banana
➤ Handful of spinach leaves
➤ 1 tablespoon flaxseeds

Instructions:

➤ Blend green tea, pineapple, banana, spinach, and flaxseeds until smooth.

Health Benefits:

➤ Green tea may contribute to lower blood pressure, and flaxseeds are rich in omega-3 fatty acids.

Preparation Time: 5 minutes

13. Veggie and Egg Breakfast Burrito

Ingredients:

- 2 whole wheat tortillas
- 2 large eggs, scrambled
- 1/2 cup black beans, drained and rinsed
- 1/4 cup diced bell peppers
- Salsa and cilantro for garnish

Instructions:

- Scramble eggs and set aside.
- Warm tortillas and fill with scrambled eggs, black beans, and bell peppers.
- Top with salsa and cilantro.

Health Benefits:

- Black beans are high in fiber and protein, supporting heart health.

Preparation Time: 15 minutes

14. Cottage Cheese and Fruit Bowl

Ingredients:

- 1 cup low-fat cottage cheese
- 1/2 cup pineapple chunks
- 1/2 cup mango slices

> 1 tablespoon sunflower seeds

Instructions:

> In a bowl, combine cottage cheese, pineapple, mango, and sunflower seeds.

Health Benefits:

> Cottage cheese provides protein and calcium, and fruits offer essential vitamins.

Preparation Time: 5 minutes

15. Walnut and Banana Overnight Oats

Ingredients:

> 1/2 cup rolled oats
> 1/2 cup low-fat milk
> 1/2 banana, mashed
> 1 tablespoon chopped walnuts
> 1 teaspoon honey

Instructions:

> Mix oats, milk, mashed banana, and chopped walnuts in a jar.
> Refrigerate overnight and drizzle honey before serving.

Health Benefits:

> ➢ Walnuts contain omega-3 fatty acids, beneficial for heart health.

Preparation Time: 5 minutes (plus overnight chilling)

Lunch Recipes:

1. Grilled Salmon with Lemon and Dill

Ingredients:

> ➢ Salmon fillets
> ➢ Lemon
> ➢ Fresh dill
> ➢ Olive oil
> ➢ Garlic
> ➢ Salt and pepper

Instructions:

> ➢ Preheat grill to medium-high heat.
> ➢ Season salmon with salt, pepper, minced garlic, and fresh dill.
> ➢ Grill salmon for 4-5 minutes per side until cooked through.
> ➢ Squeeze fresh lemon juice over the top before serving.

Health benefits:

> ➢ Salmon is rich in omega-3 fatty acids, which can help lower blood pressure and reduce inflammation.

Preparation time: 10-12 minutes

2. Quinoa and Black Bean Salad

Ingredients:

- Quinoa
- Black beans
- Cherry tomatoes
- Red onion
- Cilantro
- Lime
- Olive oil
- Salt and pepper

Instructions:

- Cook quinoa according to package instructions.
- Mix cooked quinoa with black beans, diced tomatoes, chopped red onion, and chopped cilantro.
- In a separate bowl, whisk together lime juice, olive oil, salt, and pepper.
- Toss the salad with the dressing before serving.

Health benefits:

- Quinoa is a whole grain that provides fiber and plant-based protein, contributing to heart health.

Preparation time: 20 minutes

3. Mediterranean Chickpea Salad

Ingredients:

- ➢ Chickpeas
- ➢ Cucumber
- ➢ Cherry tomatoes
- ➢ Red bell pepper
- ➢ Red onion
- ➢ Feta cheese
- ➢ Kalamata olives
- ➢ Olive oil
- ➢ Lemon juice
- ➢ Oregano
- ➢ Salt and pepper

Instructions:

- ➢ Combine chickpeas, diced cucumber, halved cherry tomatoes, chopped red bell pepper, red onion, feta cheese, and Kalamata olives in a bowl.
- ➢ In a separate bowl, whisk together olive oil, lemon juice, oregano, salt, and pepper.
- ➢ Pour the dressing over the salad and toss to combine.

Health benefits:

> ➤ This salad is rich in fiber, antioxidants, and healthy fats, supporting heart health.

Preparation time: 15 minutes

4. Vegetable Stir-Fry with Tofu

Ingredients:

- ➤ Firm tofu
- ➤ Broccoli
- ➤ Bell peppers (assorted colors)
- ➤ Carrots
- ➤ Snap peas
- ➤ Garlic
- ➤ Ginger
- ➤ Low-sodium soy sauce
- ➤ Sesame oil
- ➤ Brown rice

Instructions:

- ➤ Press tofu to remove excess water, then cut it into cubes.
- ➤ Stir-fry tofu in sesame oil until golden brown.
- ➤ Add chopped garlic and ginger, followed by broccoli, bell peppers, carrots, and snap peas.

> Stir in low-sodium soy sauce and cook until vegetables are tender-crisp.

> Serve over cooked brown rice.

Health benefits:

> Tofu provides plant-based protein, and the vegetables offer essential vitamins and minerals for heart health.

Preparation time: 25 minutes

5. Lentil and Vegetable Soup

Ingredients:

> Green or brown lentils

> Carrots

> Celery

> Onion

> Garlic

> Tomatoes

> Vegetable broth

> Cumin

> Turmeric

> Paprika

> Bay leaves

> Fresh parsley

Instructions:

> ➢ Sauté chopped onion, garlic, carrots, and celery until softened.
> ➢ Add lentils, diced tomatoes, vegetable broth, cumin, turmeric, paprika, and bay leaves.
> ➢ Simmer until lentils are tender.
> ➢ Garnish with fresh parsley before serving.

Health benefits:

> ➢ Lentils are high in fiber and protein, aiding in blood pressure regulation.

Preparation time: 30 minutes

6. Baked Chicken Breast with Herbs

Ingredients:

> ➢ Chicken breast
> ➢ Olive oil
> ➢ Garlic powder
> ➢ Onion powder
> ➢ Thyme
> ➢ Rosemary
> ➢ Paprika
> ➢ Salt and pepper

Instructions:

> Preheat the oven to 400°F (200°C).
> Rub chicken breast with olive oil and season with garlic powder, onion powder, thyme, rosemary, paprika, salt, and pepper.
> Bake until the internal temperature reaches 165°F (74°C).
> Health benefits: Lean chicken breast is a good source of protein with lower saturated fat content.

Preparation time: 25 minutes

7. Spinach and Mushroom Whole Wheat Pizza

Ingredients:

> Whole wheat pizza dough
> Tomato sauce (low-sodium)
> Mozzarella cheese (part-skim)
> Spinach
> Mushrooms
> Garlic
> Olive oil
> Red pepper flakes (optional)

Instructions:

> Roll out whole wheat pizza dough.

- ➢ Spread a thin layer of tomato sauce, top with part-skim mozzarella, spinach, mushrooms, and minced garlic.
- ➢ Drizzle with olive oil and sprinkle with red pepper flakes if desired.
- ➢ Bake according to the pizza dough instructions.

Health benefits:

- ➢ Whole wheat crust provides more fiber, and the veggies contribute to heart health.

Preparation time: Varies based on pizza dough instructions.

8. Shrimp and Vegetable Skewers

Ingredients:

- ➢ Shrimp, peeled and deveined
- ➢ Cherry tomatoes
- ➢ Zucchini
- ➢ Bell peppers (assorted colors)
- ➢ Red onion
- ➢ Olive oil
- ➢ Lemon juice
- ➢ Garlic
- ➢ Paprika
- ➢ Salt and pepper

Instructions:

> ➤ Preheat the grill or grill pan.

> ➤ Thread shrimp, cherry tomatoes, zucchini slices, bell peppers, and red onion onto skewers.

> ➤ In a bowl, mix olive oil, lemon juice, minced garlic, paprika, salt, and pepper.

> ➤ Brush the skewers with the mixture and grill until shrimp are opaque and vegetables are tender.

Health benefits:

> ➤ Shrimp is a good source of protein, and the vegetables add fiber and essential nutrients.

Preparation time: 15 minutes

9. Brown Rice and Vegetable Bowl

Ingredients:

> ➤ Brown rice

> ➤ Broccoli

> ➤ Carrots

> ➤ Edamame

> ➤ Red cabbage

> ➤ Soy sauce

> ➤ Sesame oil

> ➤ Ginger

- ➤ Garlic

- ➤ Green onions

Instructions:

- ➤ Cook brown rice according to package instructions.

- ➤ Steam broccoli, carrots, and edamame until tender-crisp.

- ➤ In a wok or pan, sauté minced garlic and ginger in sesame oil.

- ➤ Add cooked rice and steamed vegetables, toss with soy sauce, and garnish with chopped green onions.

Health benefits:

- ➤ Brown rice and vegetables provide fiber and essential nutrients for heart health.

Preparation time: 20 minutes

10. Turkey and Avocado Wrap

Ingredients:

- ➤ Whole wheat tortilla

- ➤ Turkey breast slices (low-sodium)

- ➤ Avocado

- ➤ Lettuce

- ➤ Tomato

- ➤ Greek yogurt (plain, non-fat)

- ➤ Mustard

- ➢ Salt and pepper

Instructions:

- ➢ Lay out a whole wheat tortilla and layer turkey slices, sliced avocado, lettuce, and tomato.
- ➢ Spread a mixture of Greek yogurt and mustard on the ingredients.
- ➢ Season with salt and pepper, then roll up the wrap.

Health benefits:

- ➢ Turkey is a lean protein source, and avocado provides heart-healthy monounsaturated fats.

Preparation time: 10 minutes

11. Eggplant and Tomato Stacks

Ingredients:

- ➢ Eggplant
- ➢ Tomatoes
- ➢ Mozzarella cheese (part-skim)
- ➢ Fresh basil
- ➢ Olive oil
- ➢ Balsamic vinegar
- ➢ Salt and pepper

Instructions:

> ➤ Preheat the oven to 375°F (190°C).
> ➤ Slice eggplant and tomatoes into rounds.
> ➤ Assemble stacks with eggplant, tomato, and part-skim mozzarella.
> ➤ Drizzle with olive oil and balsamic vinegar, season with salt and pepper.
> ➤ Bake until the cheese is melted and bubbly.

Health benefits:

> ➤ Eggplant is low in calories and rich in fiber, while tomatoes offer heart-protective nutrients.

Preparation time: 20 minutes

12. Chickpea and Vegetable Stir-Fry

Ingredients:

> ➤ Chickpeas
> ➤ Broccoli
> ➤ Bell peppers (assorted colors)
> ➤ Snow peas
> ➤ Carrots
> ➤ Garlic
> ➤ Ginger
> ➤ Low-sodium soy sauce

> Sesame oil

> Brown rice

Instructions:

> Sauté chickpeas, broccoli, bell peppers, snow peas, and carrots in sesame oil.

> Add minced garlic and ginger, stir-frying until vegetables are tender-crisp.

> Mix in low-sodium soy sauce.

> Serve over cooked brown rice.

Health benefits:

> Chickpeas provide protein and fiber, contributing to heart health.

Preparation time: 25 minutes

13. Tuna and White Bean Salad

Ingredients:

> Canned tuna (in water)

> Cannellini beans (canned)

> Cherry tomatoes

> Red onion

> Cucumber

> Kalamata olives

- ➢ Olive oil
- ➢ Lemon juice
- ➢ Dijon mustard
- ➢ Salt and pepper

Instructions:

- ➢ Drain canned tuna and cannellini beans.
- ➢ Combine tuna, beans, halved cherry tomatoes, diced red onion, sliced cucumber, and Kalamata olives in a bowl.
- ➢ In a separate bowl, whisk together olive oil, lemon juice, Dijon mustard, salt, and pepper.
- ➢ Toss the salad with the dressing before serving.

Health benefits:

- ➢ Tuna is rich in omega-3 fatty acids, and beans provide fiber for heart health.

Preparation time: 15 minutes

14. Sweet Potato and Black Bean Quesadillas

Ingredients:

- ➢ Sweet potatoes
- ➢ Black beans
- ➢ Whole wheat tortillas
- ➢ Cheddar cheese (reduced-fat)

- ➢ Cumin
- ➢ Paprika
- ➢ Olive oil
- ➢ Greek yogurt (plain, non-fat)

Instructions:

- ➢ Roast sweet potato cubes with cumin and paprika until tender.
- ➢ Mash black beans and spread on one half of a whole wheat tortilla.
- ➢ Top with sweet potatoes, reduced-fat cheddar cheese, and fold the tortilla.
- ➢ Cook in a skillet with olive oil until the cheese is melted.
- ➢ Serve with a side of plain, non-fat Greek yogurt.

Health benefits:

- ➢ Sweet potatoes provide potassium, and black beans offer fiber, both beneficial for heart health.

Preparation time: 30 minutes

15. Vegetable and Tofu Stir-Fry with Brown Rice

Ingredients:

- ➢ Firm tofu
- ➢ Broccoli
- ➢ Carrots

- ➢ Snap peas
- ➢ Bell peppers (assorted colors)
- ➢ Brown rice
- ➢ Low-sodium soy sauce
- ➢ Garlic
- ➢ Ginger
- ➢ Sesame oil

Instructions:

- ➢ Press tofu to remove excess water and cut into cubes.
- ➢ Stir-fry tofu, broccoli, carrots, snap peas, and bell peppers in sesame oil.
- ➢ Add minced garlic and ginger, then pour in low-sodium soy sauce.
- ➢ Serve over cooked brown rice.

Health benefits:

- ➢ Tofu provides plant-based protein, and the vegetables contribute essential nutrients for heart health.

Preparation time: 25 minutes

1: Grilled Salmon with Lemon and Herbs

Ingredients:

- Salmon fillets
- Fresh lemon
- Olive oil
- Fresh herbs (such as dill or parsley)
- Salt and pepper
- Instructions:
- Preheat the grill.
- Brush salmon fillets with olive oil, sprinkle with salt, pepper, and fresh herbs.
- Grill for 4-6 minutes per side until cooked through.
- Squeeze fresh lemon juice over the salmon before serving.

Health Benefits:

- Salmon is rich in omega-3 fatty acids, which can help lower blood pressure.

Preparation Time: 15 minutes

2: Quinoa and Vegetable Stir-Fry

Ingredients:

- Quinoa

- ➢ Mixed vegetables (bell peppers, broccoli, carrots)
- ➢ Garlic and ginger (minced)
- ➢ Low-sodium soy sauce
- ➢ Olive oil

Instructions:

- ➢ Cook quinoa according to package instructions.
- ➢ Stir-fry mixed vegetables, garlic, and ginger in olive oil.
- ➢ Add cooked quinoa and soy sauce, toss until well combined.

Health Benefits:

- ➢ Quinoa is a whole grain rich in fiber, promoting heart health.

Preparation Time: 20 minutes

3: Baked Chicken Breast with Rosemary

Ingredients:

- ➢ Chicken breasts
- ➢ Fresh rosemary
- ➢ Garlic (minced)
- ➢ Olive oil
- ➢ Lemon zest

Instructions:

- ➢ Preheat the oven.

- ➤ Rub chicken breasts with olive oil, minced garlic, rosemary, and lemon zest.

- ➤ Bake until chicken is cooked through.

Health Benefits:

- ➤ Chicken is a lean protein source, and rosemary may have blood pressure-lowering properties.

Preparation Time: 25 minutes

4: Lentil Soup

Ingredients:

- ➤ Dry lentils

- ➤ Tomatoes (canned or fresh)

- ➤ Carrots, celery, and onion (diced)

- ➤ Garlic (minced)

- ➤ Vegetable broth

- ➤ Spinach

Instructions:

- ➤ Saute garlic, onion, carrots, and celery in olive oil.

- ➤ Add lentils, tomatoes, and vegetable broth. Simmer until lentils are tender.

- ➤ Stir in fresh spinach before serving.

Health Benefits:

> Lentils are high in potassium, fiber, and protein, supporting heart health.

Preparation Time: 30 minutes

5: Shrimp and Vegetable Skewers

Ingredients:

> Shrimp (peeled and deveined)
> Bell peppers, zucchini, cherry tomatoes
> Olive oil
> Lemon juice
> Garlic powder and paprika

Instructions:

> Thread shrimp and vegetables onto skewers.
> Brush with olive oil, lemon juice, and sprinkle with garlic powder and paprika.
> Grill until shrimp are opaque and vegetables are tender.

Health Benefits:

> Shrimp is a low-calorie protein source, and vegetables provide essential nutrients.

Preparation Time: 15 minutes

6: Spinach and Feta Stuffed Chicken Breast

Ingredients:

- ➢ Chicken breasts
- ➢ Fresh spinach
- ➢ Feta cheese
- ➢ Garlic (minced)
- ➢ Olive oil

Instructions:

- ➢ Butterfly chicken breasts.
- ➢ Saute spinach and garlic in olive oil until wilted. Stuff chicken with the mixture and feta.
- ➢ Bake until chicken is cooked through.

Health Benefits:

- ➢ Spinach is rich in potassium and feta provides calcium, supporting overall heart health.

Preparation Time: 30 minutes

7: Brown Rice and Black Bean Bowl

Ingredients:

- ➢ Brown rice
- ➢ Black beans (canned or cooked)
- ➢ Avocado, corn, and cherry tomatoes

> Cilantro and lime

Instructions:

> Cook brown rice according to package instructions.
> Combine rice, black beans, diced avocado, corn, and cherry tomatoes.
> Garnish with chopped cilantro and a squeeze of lime.

Health Benefits:

> Brown rice and black beans are high in fiber, aiding heart health.

Preparation Time: 25 minutes

8: Baked Cod with Mediterranean Salsa

Ingredients:

> Cod fillets
> Tomatoes, olives, and red onion (diced)
> Fresh parsley
> Olive oil
> Balsamic vinegar

Instructions:

> Preheat the oven.
> Season cod with olive oil and bake until flaky.

> Mix diced tomatoes, olives, red onion, parsley, and a splash of
balsamic vinegar for salsa.

Health Benefits:

> Cod is a lean protein, and Mediterranean salsa adds heart-
healthy fats.

Preparation Time: 20 minutes

9: Chickpea and Vegetable Curry

Ingredients:

> Chickpeas (canned or cooked)
> Mixed vegetables (bell peppers, cauliflower, peas)
> Coconut milk
> Curry powder, turmeric, and cumin
> Garlic and ginger (minced)

Instructions:

> Saute garlic, ginger, and vegetables in coconut oil.
> Add chickpeas, coconut milk, and spices. Simmer until
vegetables are tender.

Health Benefits:

> Chickpeas are rich in fiber, and curry spices may have anti-
inflammatory properties.

Preparation Time: 30 minutes

10: Turkey and Sweet Potato Chili

Ingredients:

- Ground turkey
- Sweet potatoes (diced)
- Black beans (canned or cooked)
- Diced tomatoes (canned or fresh)
- Chili powder, cumin, and paprika

Instructions:

- Brown ground turkey in a pot.
- Add sweet potatoes, black beans, diced tomatoes, and spices. Simmer until sweet potatoes are cooked.

Health Benefits:

- Turkey is a lean protein, and sweet potatoes provide potassium.

Preparation Time: 40 minutes

11: Eggplant and Tomato Stacks

Ingredients:

- Eggplant
- Tomatoes

- Mozzarella cheese
- Fresh basil
- Balsamic glaze

Instructions:

- Slice eggplant and tomatoes.
- Assemble stacks with mozzarella and fresh basil.
- Bake until cheese is melted. Drizzle with balsamic glaze before serving.

Health Benefits:

- Eggplant and tomatoes are rich in antioxidants.

Preparation Time: 25 minutes

12: Whole Wheat Pasta with Tomato and Garlic Sauce

Ingredients:

- Whole wheat pasta
- Tomatoes (canned or fresh)
- Garlic (minced)
- Olive oil
- Fresh basil

Instructions:

- Cook whole wheat pasta according to package instructions.
- Saute minced garlic in olive oil, add tomatoes, and simmer.

➢ Toss pasta with the sauce and garnish with fresh basil.

Health Benefits:

➢ Whole wheat pasta provides more fiber than traditional pasta.

Preparation Time: 20 minutes

13: Vegetable and Tofu Stir-Fry

Ingredients:

➢ Tofu

➢ Broccoli, bell peppers, and snap peas

➢ Soy sauce and sesame oil

➢ Ginger and garlic (minced)

Instructions:

➢ Press and cube tofu.

➢ Stir-fry tofu and vegetables in sesame oil, soy sauce, ginger, and garlic until vegetables are tender.

Health Benefits:

➢ Tofu is a plant-based protein, and vegetables provide essential nutrients.

Preparation Time: 25 minutes

14: Greek Salad with Grilled Chicken

Ingredients:

- Chicken breasts
- Romaine lettuce, cucumber, cherry tomatoes, and feta cheese
- Kalamata olives
- Greek dressing

Instructions:

- Grill chicken until fully cooked.
- Assemble salad with chopped lettuce, cucumber, cherry tomatoes, feta, and olives.
- Top with sliced grilled chicken and drizzle with Greek dressing.

Health Benefits:

- A Mediterranean-style salad with lean protein and heart-healthy fats.

Preparation Time: 30 minutes

15: Cauliflower and Chickpea Curry

Ingredients:

- Cauliflower florets
- Chickpeas (canned or cooked)
- Coconut milk

- ➢ Curry powder, turmeric, and cumin
- ➢ Garlic and ginger (minced)

Instructions:

- ➢ Saute garlic, ginger, cauliflower, and chickpeas in coconut oil.
- ➢ Add coconut milk and spices. Simmer until cauliflower is tender.

Health Benefits:

- ➢ Cauliflower is low in calories and rich in vitamins, and chickpeas provide fiber and protein.

Preparation Time: 35 minutes

Snack Recipes:

1. Avocado and Tomato Salsa

Ingredients:

- ➢ 2 ripe avocados, diced
- ➢ 1 cup cherry tomatoes, halved
- ➢ 1/4 cup red onion, finely chopped
- ➢ 2 tablespoons fresh cilantro, chopped
- ➢ 1 lime, juiced
- ➢ Salt and pepper to taste

Instructions:

- In a bowl, combine avocados, tomatoes, red onion, and cilantro.
- Squeeze lime juice over the mixture and season with salt and pepper.
- Gently toss ingredients until well combined.

Health Benefits:

- Rich in potassium and heart-healthy monounsaturated fats.

Preparation Time: 10 minutes

2. Greek Yogurt and Berry Parfait

Ingredients:

- 1 cup Greek yogurt
- 1/2 cup mixed berries (blueberries, strawberries, raspberries)
- 2 tablespoons honey
- 1/4 cup granola

Instructions:

- In a glass, layer Greek yogurt, mixed berries, and granola.
- Drizzle honey over the top.

Health Benefits:

- High in antioxidants, fiber, and probiotics.

Preparation Time: 5 minutes

3. Cucumber and Hummus Bites

Ingredients:

- 1 cucumber, sliced
- 1/2 cup hummus
- Cherry tomatoes for garnish
- Fresh parsley, chopped

Instructions:

- Spread hummus on cucumber slices.
- Top each slice with a cherry tomato and sprinkle with fresh parsley.

Health Benefits:

- Low in sodium, hydrating, and provides healthy fats.

Preparation Time: 10 minutes

4. Baked Sweet Potato Chips

Ingredients:

- 2 sweet potatoes, thinly sliced
- 2 tablespoons olive oil
- 1 teaspoon smoked paprika
- 1/2 teaspoon sea salt

Instructions:

> Preheat oven to 400°F (200°C).
> Toss sweet potato slices with olive oil, smoked paprika, and sea salt.
> Arrange in a single layer on a baking sheet and bake for 20-25 minutes or until crispy.

Health Benefits:

> High in potassium and fiber, lower in sodium than store-bought chips.

Preparation Time: 25 minutes

5. Quinoa Salad Cups

Ingredients:

> 1 cup cooked quinoa
> 1/2 cup cucumber, diced
> 1/2 cup cherry tomatoes, quartered
> 1/4 cup feta cheese, crumbled
> 2 tablespoons olive oil
> Fresh lemon juice, to taste

Instructions:

> In a bowl, mix quinoa, cucumber, tomatoes, and feta cheese.

- ➢ Drizzle with olive oil and lemon juice, toss until well combined.
- ➢ Serve in small lettuce cups or on cucumber slices.

Health Benefits:

- ➢ Quinoa is rich in protein and fiber, promoting heart health.

Preparation Time: 15 minutes

6. Edamame and Sea Salt

Ingredients:

- ➢ 1 cup edamame, steamed
- ➢ Sea salt, to taste
- ➢ Instructions:
- ➢ Steam edamame according to package instructions.
- ➢ Sprinkle with sea salt and toss to coat.

Health Benefits:

- ➢ Edamame is a good source of soy protein and low in sodium.

Preparation Time: 5 minutes

7. Almond and Berry Smoothie Bowl

Ingredients:

- ➢ 1 cup almond milk
- ➢ 1/2 cup mixed berries (strawberries, blueberries, raspberries)

- ➢ 1 banana, frozen
- ➢ 2 tablespoons almond butter
- ➢ Toppings: sliced almonds, chia seeds, fresh berries

Instructions:

- ➢ Blend almond milk, mixed berries, frozen banana, and almond butter until smooth.
- ➢ Pour into a bowl and top with sliced almonds, chia seeds, and fresh berries.

Health Benefits:

- ➢ Almonds are rich in magnesium, and berries provide antioxidants.

Preparation Time: 5 minutes

8. Spinach and Artichoke Dip

Ingredients:

- ➢ 1 cup Greek yogurt
- ➢ 1 cup fresh spinach, chopped
- ➢ 1/2 cup artichoke hearts, drained and chopped
- ➢ 1/4 cup Parmesan cheese, grated
- ➢ 1 clove garlic, minced
- ➢ Whole grain pita bread or vegetable sticks for dipping

Instructions:

- ➤ In a bowl, mix Greek yogurt, spinach, artichoke hearts, Parmesan, and minced garlic.
- ➤ Refrigerate for at least 30 minutes before serving.
- ➤ Serve with whole grain pita or vegetable sticks.

Health Benefits:

- ➤ Spinach is high in potassium, and Greek yogurt provides protein.

Preparation Time: 10 minutes

9. Mango Salsa with Whole Grain Tortilla Chips

Ingredients:

- ➤ 1 ripe mango, diced
- ➤ 1/2 red bell pepper, diced
- ➤ 1/4 cup red onion, finely chopped
- ➤ 1 jalapeño, seeded and minced
- ➤ 2 tablespoons fresh cilantro, chopped
- ➤ Juice of 1 lime
- ➤ Whole grain tortilla chips

Instructions:

- ➤ In a bowl, combine mango, red bell pepper, red onion, jalapeño, cilantro, and lime juice.

➢ Refrigerate for at least 15 minutes before serving with whole grain tortilla chips.

Health Benefits:

➢ Mangoes contain potassium, and whole grain chips offer fiber.

Preparation Time: 15 minutes

10. Roasted Chickpeas

Ingredients:

➢ 1 can (15 oz) chickpeas, drained and rinsed
➢ 1 tablespoon olive oil
➢ 1 teaspoon smoked paprika
➢ 1/2 teaspoon cumin
➢ 1/2 teaspoon garlic powder
➢ Sea salt, to taste

Instructions:

➢ Preheat oven to 400°F (200°C).
➢ Toss chickpeas with olive oil, smoked paprika, cumin, garlic powder, and sea salt.
➢ Roast for 20-25 minutes or until crispy.

Health Benefits:

➢ Chickpeas are high in fiber and protein, supporting heart health.

Preparation Time: 25 minutes

11. Berry and Almond Oat Bars

Ingredients:

- 1 cup rolled oats
- 1/2 cup almond butter
- 1/4 cup honey
- 1/2 cup mixed berries (blueberries, raspberries)
- 1/4 cup almonds, chopped

Instructions:

- In a bowl, mix rolled oats, almond butter, and honey until well combined.
- Fold in mixed berries and chopped almonds.
- Press the mixture into a lined pan and refrigerate for at least 2 hours before cutting into bars.

Health Benefits:

- Oats are high in soluble fiber, almonds provide healthy fats, and berries are rich in antioxidants.

Preparation Time: 10 minutes (plus refrigeration time)

12. Vegetable Stuffed Whole Wheat Pita Pockets

Ingredients:

- Whole wheat pita pockets
- Hummus
- 1 cup mixed vegetables (cucumber, cherry tomatoes, bell peppers), diced

Instructions:

- Cut the top off each pita pocket to create an opening.
- Spread hummus inside the pockets and stuff with mixed vegetables.

Health Benefits:

- Whole wheat is high in fiber, and vegetables provide essential nutrients.

Preparation Time: 10 minutes

13. Salmon and Avocado Roll-ups

Ingredients:

- Smoked salmon slices
- 1 ripe avocado, sliced
- Greek yogurt (optional for dipping)

Instructions:

> Lay out smoked salmon slices.
> Place a slice of avocado on each salmon slice and roll it up.
> Secure with toothpicks and serve with a side of Greek yogurt if desired.

Health Benefits:

> Salmon is rich in omega-3 fatty acids, and avocados provide potassium.

Preparation Time: 15 minutes

14. Whole Grain Crackers with Tuna Salad

Ingredients:

> Whole grain crackers
> 1 can (5 oz) tuna, drained
> 1/4 cup Greek yogurt
> 1/2 celery stalk, finely chopped
> 1 tablespoon Dijon mustard
> Salt and pepper to taste

Instructions:

> In a bowl, mix tuna, Greek yogurt, celery, Dijon mustard, salt, and pepper.
> Spoon the tuna salad onto whole grain crackers.

Health Benefits:

> ➤ Tuna is a good source of omega-3s, and whole grains provide fiber.

Preparation Time: 10 minutes

15. Green Tea and Mixed Nuts

Ingredients:

> ➤ Mixed nuts (almonds, walnuts, pistachios)
> ➤ Green tea (unsweetened)

Instructions:

> ➤ Measure a small serving of mixed nuts.
> ➤ Brew a cup of green tea and enjoy it with the mixed nuts.

Health Benefits:

> ➤ Nuts contain healthy fats, and green tea is rich in antioxidants.

Preparation Time: 5 minutes

BONUS

Heart Healthy Recipes:

1: Grilled Salmon with Lemon and Dill

Ingredients:

> ➤ Salmon fillets

- ➢ Fresh lemon
- ➢ Fresh dill
- ➢ Olive oil
- ➢ Salt and pepper

Instructions:

- ➢ Preheat the grill.
- ➢ Season salmon with salt, pepper, and olive oil.
- ➢ Grill salmon for 4-5 minutes per side until it flakes easily.
- ➢ Squeeze fresh lemon juice over the top and sprinkle with chopped dill.

Health Benefits:

- ➢ Rich in omega-3 fatty acids for heart health.
- ➢ High in protein.

Preparation Time: 10-12 minutes

2: Quinoa and Vegetable Stir-Fry

Ingredients:

- ➢ Quinoa
- ➢ Mixed vegetables (broccoli, bell peppers, carrots)
- ➢ Soy sauce
- ➢ Garlic
- ➢ Olive oil

Instructions:

- ➢ Cook quinoa according to package instructions.
- ➢ Sauté garlic in olive oil, add chopped vegetables, and stir-fry.
- ➢ Mix in cooked quinoa and soy sauce until well combined.

Health Benefits:

- ➢ Quinoa provides protein and fiber.
- ➢ Vegetables offer essential vitamins and minerals.

Preparation Time: 20 minutes

3: Baked Chicken Breast with Herbs

Ingredients:

- ➢ Chicken breasts
- ➢ Fresh herbs (rosemary, thyme, parsley)
- ➢ Garlic
- ➢ Olive oil
- ➢ Salt and pepper

Instructions:

- ➢ Preheat the oven.
- ➢ Rub chicken with olive oil, minced garlic, chopped herbs, salt, and pepper.
- ➢ Bake until the internal temperature reaches 165°F.

Health Benefits:

- ➤ Lean protein for muscle health.
- ➤ Herbs add flavor without excess salt.

Preparation Time: 25-30 minutes

4: Lentil and Vegetable Soup

Ingredients:

- ➤ Lentils
- ➤ Mixed vegetables (carrots, celery, tomatoes)
- ➤ Vegetable broth
- ➤ Onion
- ➤ Garlic

Instructions:

- ➤ Sauté onion and garlic in a pot.
- ➤ Add vegetables, lentils, and vegetable broth.
- ➤ Simmer until lentils are tender.

Health Benefits:

- ➤ High in fiber and plant-based protein.
- ➤ Supports heart health.

Preparation Time: 40 minutes

5: Spinach and Berry Salad with Balsamic Vinaigrette

Ingredients:

- Fresh spinach
- Mixed berries (strawberries, blueberries, raspberries)
- Feta cheese
- Balsamic vinaigrette

Instructions:

- Toss fresh spinach with berries and crumbled feta.
- Drizzle with balsamic vinaigrette.

Health Benefits:

- Berries provide antioxidants.
- Spinach is rich in vitamins and minerals.

Preparation Time: 15 minutes

6: Whole Grain Pasta with Tomato and Basil

Ingredients:

- Whole grain pasta
- Fresh tomatoes
- Fresh basil
- Garlic
- Olive oil

Instructions:

> ➤ Cook pasta according to package instructions.
> ➤ Sauté garlic in olive oil, add chopped tomatoes and basil.
> ➤ Toss cooked pasta with the tomato mixture.

Health Benefits:

> ➤ Whole grain pasta for added fiber.
> ➤ Tomatoes and basil offer vitamins and antioxidants.

Preparation Time: 15-20 minutes

7: Greek Yogurt Parfait with Mixed Nuts and Honey

Ingredients:

> ➤ Greek yogurt
> ➤ Mixed nuts (almonds, walnuts)
> ➤ Honey
> ➤ Fresh berries

Instructions:

> ➤ Layer Greek yogurt with mixed nuts and fresh berries.
> ➤ Drizzle with honey.

Health Benefits:

> ➤ Greek yogurt provides protein and probiotics.
> ➤ Nuts offer heart-healthy fats.

Preparation Time: 10 minutes

8: Oven-Roasted Vegetables

Ingredients:

- ➤ Assorted vegetables (bell peppers, zucchini, cherry tomatoes)
- ➤ Olive oil
- ➤ Garlic powder
- ➤ Italian seasoning

Instructions:

- ➤ Preheat the oven.
- ➤ Toss vegetables with olive oil and seasonings.
- ➤ Roast until vegetables are tender.

Health Benefits:

- ➤ Vegetables are rich in vitamins and minerals.
- ➤ Olive oil provides healthy fats.

Preparation Time: 25 minutes

9: Turkey and Veggie Lettuce Wraps

Ingredients:

- ➤ Ground turkey
- ➤ Lettuce leaves
- ➤ Mixed vegetables (bell peppers, carrots, mushrooms)

- ➤ Soy sauce
- ➤ Ginger

Instructions:

- ➤ Brown ground turkey in a pan.
- ➤ Add chopped vegetables, soy sauce, and ginger.
- ➤ Spoon the mixture into lettuce leaves.

Health Benefits:

- ➤ Lean protein from turkey.
- ➤ Low-carb option with plenty of veggies.

Preparation Time: 20 minutes

10: Berry Smoothie with Flaxseeds

Ingredients:

- ➤ Mixed berries (strawberries, blueberries, raspberries)
- ➤ Greek yogurt
- ➤ Almond milk
- ➤ Flaxseeds

Instructions:

- ➤ Blend berries, Greek yogurt, almond milk, and flaxseeds until smooth.
- ➤ Adjust thickness with more almond milk if needed.

Health Benefits:

- ➤ Berries are rich in antioxidants.
- ➤ Flaxseeds provide omega-3 fatty acids.

Preparation Time: 5 minutes

CONCLUSION

In concluding this High Blood Pressure Cookbook for Beginners, we embark on a journey that celebrates not only the joy of cooking but also the profound impact it can have on our cardiovascular well-being. The recipes shared in this cookbook are not just culinary creations; they are gateways to a heart-healthy lifestyle.

As we've explored the art of crafting meals that nurture our bodies and minds, it's essential to recognize the power we hold in our hands — the power to make choices that positively influence our blood pressure and overall health. Each ingredient, every cooking method, and the mindful selection of nutrients contribute to the symphony of well-being that resonates within us.

From vibrant salads to wholesome soups, from succulent grilled proteins to nutrient-packed smoothies, the recipes provided here aim to inspire and guide you towards a flavorful journey of heart-healthy living. By embracing these culinary delights, you are not just fostering good eating habits but also laying the foundation for a healthier, happier life.

Remember, the essence of this cookbook extends beyond the kitchen. It's about making conscious choices, relishing the diversity of fresh, nutrient-rich ingredients, and savoring the flavors that nature graciously provides.

As you continue to explore the realm of heart-healthy cooking, consider it a personal commitment to the well-being of your heart and the hearts of those you care about.

In closing, let the recipes within these pages serve as a starting point for your own culinary adventures. May your kitchen be a place of creativity, nourishment, and love, fostering not only delicious meals but also a heart that beats strong and steady.

Here's to your heart — to health, happiness, and the delightful journey of heart-healthy Preparation!